2.50

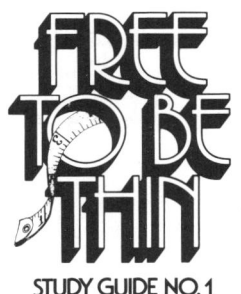

STUDY GUIDE NO. 1

This is a study guide to be used along with the official Overeaters Victorious study manual, *Free To Be Thin*, by Marie Chapian. For maximum benefit of this study there is a set of teaching tapes titled *Free To Be Thin* by Neva Coyle also available. See last page for further information.

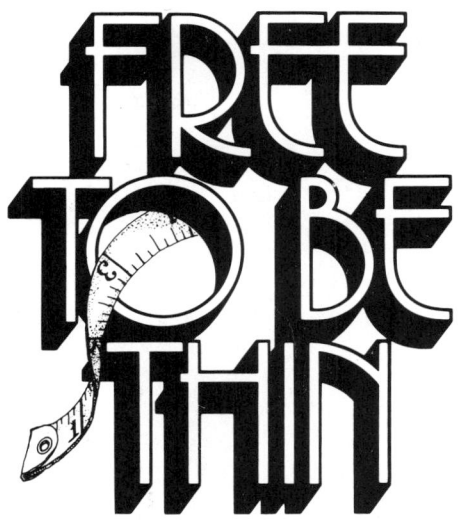

FREE TO BE THIN

STUDY GUIDE NO. 1

GETTING STARTED:

A SUCCESSFUL WEIGHT-LOSS PLAN WHICH LINKS LEARNING HOW TO EAT & HOW TO LIVE.

NEVA COYLE

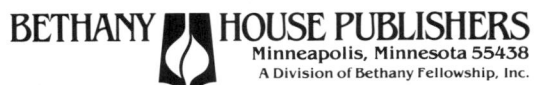

BETHANY HOUSE PUBLISHERS
Minneapolis, Minnesota 55438
A Division of Bethany Fellowship, Inc.

All Scripture references are taken from the New American Standard Bible unless otherwise noted.

*Free To Be Thin Study Guide No. 1—
Getting Started*

ISBN 0-87123-163-8

Copyright © 1980
Neva Coyle
All Rights Reserved

Published by Bethany House Publishers
6820 Auto Club Road, Minneapolis, Minnesota 55438

Printed in the United States of America

A Note from Neva

Welcome to the most exciting time of your life. From my own experience and the experience of others, I know that you are on the threshold of a miracle in your life—a miracle above and beyond anything you could ask or think. That is God's way.

We at OVEREATERS VICTORIOUS are available to help you in any way we can. The first thing I have done is to make this Study Guide available to you.

When you have finished *Free To Be Thin*, there are succeeding series should you desire to continue. A form is included in the back of this booklet to receive further information.

In preparation for each lesson you will find for your use a "Basic Journal Sheet." I suggest using the sheet in your daily quiet time prior to completing the corresponding lesson.

Because of Jesus,

Neva Coyle

Contents

Preparation for Lesson One 11
Lesson One—OBJECTIVES 14
Recommended Diet Guideline—THE SIMPLE WAY TO EAT 16
FOOD FACTS 18
Preparation for Lesson Two 20
Lesson Two—THE BEGINNING 23
Preparation for Lesson Three 27
Lesson Three—OUR GOAL 30
Preparation for Lesson Four 33
Lesson Four—DECIDING TO OBEY 36
Preparation for Lesson Five 39
Lesson Five—THE BENEFITS OF THE LAW 42
Preparation for Lesson Six 46
Lesson Six—WALKING IN HIS WILL 49
Preparation for Lesson Seven 53
Lesson Seven—POSITION AND PRACTICE 56

"But examine everything carefully; hold fast to that which is good."—1 Thessalonians 5:21

"He who began a good work in you will perfect it until the day of Christ Jesus."—Philippians 1:6

How to use this book:
In order for you to receive the maximum benefit from this study, there is a very simple procedure for you to follow. Each day, preferably in the morning, read the scriptures listed in one section of the Basic Journal Sheet. You can complete the lesson portion which corresponds with that assigned passage or you can leave the lesson until the latter part of the week and do the lesson all at once. After completing the Basic Journal Sheet and also the lesson in this book, then listen to the FTBT tape which corresponds with this lesson.

Very simply stated: first, the Basic Journal Sheet; second, the lesson itself; and third, listen to the tape.

It will be very tempting to run ahead and try to get as much of the material covered as quickly as possible. However, it is not covering the material which will help you lose weight but taking the time necessary to have the teaching become part of you. Don't hurry, and don't worry about losing interest—it is discipline you are after and that will come. Give yourself time and be patient with your progress. We are after *lasting* results, not fast results which don't last.

Preparation for Lesson One

BASIC JOURNAL SHEET

1ST DAY _____ TIME _____ REFERENCE: Deut. 29:9-13
God is impressing on me: | I've shared with the Lord . . .

Thoughts I'm having today: _____

2ND DAY _____ TIME _____ REFERENCE: Deut. 30:11-14
God is impressing on me: | I've shared with the Lord . . .

Thoughts I'm having today: _____

3RD DAY _____ TIME ____ REFERENCE: Deut. 30:15-18
God is impressing on me: | I've shared with the Lord . . .

Thoughts I'm having today: _____

4TH DAY _____ TIME ____ REFERENCE: Deut. 30:19-20
God is impressing on me: | I've shared with the Lord . . .

Thoughts I'm having today: _____

5TH DAY _____ TIME ____ REFERENCE: 1 Cor. 6:20; Matt. 5:16
God is impressing on me: | I've shared with the Lord . . .

Thoughts I'm having today: _____

6TH DAY _____ TIME ____ REFERENCE: Acts 10:36; Rom. 6:16
God is impressing on me: | I've shared with the Lord . . .

Thoughts I'm having today: _____
_____
_____

7TH DAY _____ TIME ____ REFERENCE: Gal. 5:22-23
God is impressing on me: | I've shared with the Lord . . .

Thoughts I'm having today: _____
_____
_____

WEEKLY EVALUATION

What principles has the Lord taught me this week? _____

How can I be more faithful in honoring the Lord next week? _____

What changes am I seeing in my attitude towards:
    Food? _____
    God? _____
    Others? _____

LESSON ONE

Introduction

IT'S UP TO YOU

Date today_____Weight today_____

Just before God gave Moses the law, He went through a series of statements about the importance of a covenant. Let's look at what God was expecting of the people once He gave them the law.

The promise of prosperity or success is found in Deut. 29:9-13 (New American Standard Version).

Vs. 9: *"So keep the words of this covenant to do them, that you may prosper in all that you do."*

Vss. 10-13: *"You stand today . . . before the Lord your God . . . that you may enter into the covenant with the Lord your God, and into His oath which the Lord your God is making with you today, in order that He may establish you today as His people and that He may be your God, just as He spoke to you and as He swore to your fathers, to Abraham, Isaac, and Jacob."*

This is what we have to do today. We have to enter into a covenant with God to lose weight *His way*. We all know that our own methods for losing weight have failed and disappointed us. But God will never disappoint us. Right now you can have the assurance that God is going to join with you and not only encourage you along the way to thinness but also show you the way to do it. We at OV do not say, "Here is our plan, Lord. Bless it." But rather, "What is your plan, Lord? Teach us your ways."

When we approach God on His terms, seeking His ways, asking His guidance, He then speaks to us words of comfort and encouragement.

Objectives

Deut. 30:11: *"For this commandment which I command you today is _____ too difficult for you, nor is it _____ _____ _____."*

Deut. 30:14: *"But the word is very _____ you, in _____ _____ and in your _____, that you _____ _____ _____."*

Vs. 15: *"See, I have set before you today life and prosperity, and death and adversity; in that I command you today to love the Lord your God, to walk in _____ ways and to keep _____ commandments and _____ statutes and _____ judgments, that you may live and multiply, and that the Lord your God may bless you in the land where you are entering to possess it."*

You see, the promise of being thin God's way is our promised land. But the Word goes on:

Vss. 17-18: *"But if your heart _____ _____ and you will not _____, but are drawn away and worship other gods and serve them, I declare to you today that you shall surely perish. You shall not prolong your days in the land where you are crossing the Jordan to enter and possess it."*

How can you lose your promise of being thin? _____

In verse 19, God sets before us today a choice. What is it? _____

Statistics show us that overweight bodies live shorter lives than thin bodies. We really do have before us the choice of life and death.

The scriptures urge us to choose _____.

How do we choose life?

Vs. 20: *"By loving the Lord your God, by _____ _____ _____, and by _____ _____ _____ _____."*

The overall objectives of OV are:
1. To glorify and lift up Jesus (1 Cor. 6:20; Matt. 5:16).
2. To put Jesus in the position of Lordship over every area of our lives (Acts 10:36, NASB; Col. 1:18).
3. To bring the body into control by retraining the flesh in the power of the Spirit (Gal. 5:22-23).
4. To teach you to eat in obedience to the Holy Spirit, not learn to diet (Rom. 6:16).

When you join OV you make a commitment. This is not a thing to be taken lightly, but a commitment that should be carefully settled in prayer. Our program is planned on a quarterly basis, and the commitment you make at this point is threefold:

1. *Attendance* at your chapter or group meeting (or, if you are studying as an individual, weekly completion of each lesson).

You cannot learn to walk in a disciplined life with God spasmodically. You must stay faithful to a schedule if you are to benefit fully from the lessons. There might be days of discouragement and a feeling that you'll never make it, but these days are temporary. You can best work through these feelings and phases if you remain faithful and regular in your schedule.

2. *Homework assignments* completed on a regular weekly schedule.

You will get the best results if you give regular, daily attention to the homework assignments.

3. *Immediate application* of new truths learned.

We are assuming new responsibilities to walk in the principles we learn.

"If we walk in the _____ as He Himself is in the _____, we have _____ with one another, and the _____ of Jesus His Son _____ us from all _____."

This passage in 1 John 1:7 shows us that as the light God gives us illumines our pathway a little more, we must progress. Don't worry about all you don't understand; walk in what you do understand.

ASSIGNMENT:

1. In preparation for the next lesson: Use the Basic Journal Sheet: Lesson Two. Purchase a spiral or loose-leaf notebook for additional entries.
2. Use the Calorie Account Sheet to record the food you eat and begin to record the calorie values—NOW!
3. In preparation for the next lesson, read the Introduction and chapters 1 and 2 in *Free To Be Thin* by Marie Chapian.

RECOMMENDED DIET GUIDELINE

"The Simple Way to Eat"

(For most women and small-frame men)

BREAKFAST:

High Vitamin C fruit
Protein food (choose one)
  2 oz. cottage or pot cheese
  1 oz. hard cheese
  1 egg
  2 oz. cooked or canned fish
  8 oz. skimmed milk
Bread or cereal, whole grain (choose one)
  1 slice whole grain bread
  3/4 cup ready-to-eat cereal
  1/2 cup cooked cereal
Beverage

LUNCH:

Protein food (choose one)
  2 oz. fish, poultry or lean meat
  4 oz. cottage or pot cheese
  2 oz. hard cheese
  1 egg
  2 level tablespoons peanut butter
Bread—2 slices whole grain
Vegetables—raw or cooked, except
  potato or substitute
Fruit—1 serving
Beverage

(For most men and large-frame women)

BREAKFAST:

High Vitamin C fruit
Protein food (choose one)
  2 oz. cottage or pot cheese
  1 oz. hard cheese
  1 egg
  2 oz. cooked or canned fish
  8 oz. skimmed milk
Bread or cereal, whole grain (choose one)
  2 slices whole grain bread
  1 1/2 cups ready-to-eat cereal
  1/2 cup cooked cereal
Beverage

LUNCH:

Protein food (choose one)
  2 oz. fish, poultry or lean meat
  4 oz. cottage or pot cheese
  2 oz. hard cheese
  1 egg
  2 level tablespoons peanut butter
Bread—2 slices whole grain
Vegetables—raw or cooked, except
  potato or substitute
Fruit—1 serving
Beverage

DINNER:

Protein food (choose one)
 4 oz. cooked fish, poultry or lean meat
Vegetables—cooked and raw
 High Vitamin A—choose from Food Facts
 Potato or substitute from Food Facts
 Other vegetables—you may eat responsibly
Fruit—1 serving
Beverage

OTHER DAILY FOODS:

Fat—choose 3 from Food Facts
Milk—2 cups (8 oz. each) skimmed or substitute from Food Facts

DINNER:

Protein food (choose one)
 6 oz. cooked fish, poultry or lean meat
Vegetables—cooked and raw
 High Vitamin A—choose from Food Facts
 Potato or substitute from Food Facts
 Other vegetables—you may eat responsibly
Fruit—1 serving
Beverage

OTHER DAILY FOODS:

Fat—choose 6 from Food Facts
Milk—2 cups (8 oz. each) skimmed or substitute from Food Facts

REMEMBER TO MEASURE QUANTITIES OF EACH SERVING AND ACCOUNT FOR EVERY CALORIE!!

Food Facts

LIMIT THESE PROTEIN FOODS:
Lean beef, pork, lamb to 1 pound per week total
Eggs to 4 per week
Hard cheese to 4 oz. per week

HIGH VITAMIN C FRUITS (no sugar added)
1 medium orange	1/2 medium cantaloupe	1 cup strawberries
1/2 medium mango	1/2 medium grapefruit	1 large tangerine
4 oz. orange/grapefruit juice		8 oz. tomato juice

OTHER FRUITS (no sugar added)
1 medium apple or peach	1 small banana or pear	1/4 lb. cherries or grapes
1/2 cup pineapple	1/2 cup berries	2-3 apricots/prunes/plums
1/2 round slice watermelon (1"x10")	1/2 small honeydew melon	2 tablespoons raisins

HIGH VITAMIN A VEGETABLES
Broccoli	Escarole	Pumpkin
Carrots	Mustard greens, collards and other leafy greens	Winter squash
Chicory		Watercress

POTATO OR SUBSTITUTE
1 medium potato   1 small ear corn
1 small sweet potato or yam 1/2 cup corn or green lima beans, peas
1/2 cup cooked brown rice   1/2 cup cooked dry beans, peas, lentils

FAT
1 teaspoon safflower oil   1 teaspoon margarine with liquid vegetable oil listed first
1 teaspoon mayonnaise   on label of ingredients
2 teaspoons French dressing 1 teaspoon butter

SKIMMED MILK OR SUBSTITUTE
2 cups (8 oz. each) buttermilk
2/3 cup non-fat dry milk solids
1 cup (8 oz.) evaporated skimmed milk

YOU MAY DRINK:
Coffee   Tea   Water   Club Soda   Bouillon   Consomme

YOU MAY USE:
Salt   Pepper   Herbs   Spices   Lemon/Lime   Horseradish   Vinegar

YOU MAY EAT FREELY:

Asparagus	Collards	Romaine lettuce
Green and wax beans	Cucumber	Spinach
Broccoli	Dandelion greens	Summer squash
Brussel sprouts	Escarole	Swiss chard
Carrots	Kale	Tomato
Cauliflower	Lettuce	Turnip greens
Celery	Mustard Greens	Watercress
Chicory	Parsley	

TRY TO AVOID:

Bacon, fatty meats, sausage	Cream—sweet and sour	Gelatin desserts, puddings (both diet and sugar sweetened)
Beer, liquor, wines	Cream cheese, non-dairy cream substitutes	
Butter, margarine (other than described above)	French fried potatoes, potato chips	Gravies and sauces
Cakes, cookies, crackers		Honey, jams, jellies, sugar and syrup
Doughnuts, pastries, pies	Pizza, popcorn, pretzels and similar snacks	
Candy, chocolates, nuts		Ice cream, ices, ice milk, sherbets, frozen yogurt
Whole milk	Olives	
Muffins, pancakes, waffles	Soda (both diet and sugar sweetened)	Spaghetti, macaroni, noodles
Yogurt (fruit-flavored)		

Preparation for Lesson Two

BASIC JOURNAL SHEET

1ST DAY _____ TIME ____ REFERENCE: 2 Cor. 5:1-10 (9-10)
God is impressing on me: | I've shared with the Lord . . .

- -

Thoughts I'm having today: _____

2ND DAY _____ TIME ____ REFERENCE: 1 Sam. 15:22
God is impressing on me: | I've shared with the Lord . . .

- -

Thoughts I'm having today: _____

3RD DAY _____ TIME ____ REFERENCE: Phil. 2:1-11
God is impressing on me: | I've shared with the Lord . . .

Thoughts I'm having today: _____

4TH DAY _____ TIME ____ REFERENCE: Phil. 2:12-18, 3:18-19
God is impressing on me: | I've shared with the Lord . . .

Thoughts I'm having today: _____

5TH DAY _____ TIME ____ REFERENCE: Phil. 1:6
God is impressing on me: | I've shared with the Lord . . .

Thoughts I'm having today: _____

6TH DAY _____ TIME ____ REFERENCE: 1 Cor. 3:10-17 (16)
God is impressing on me: | I've shared with the Lord . . .

Thoughts I'm having today: _____

7TH DAY _____ TIME ____ REFERENCE: Haggai 1:8, 2:3-9
God is impressing on me: | I've shared with the Lord . . .

Thoughts I'm having today: _____

WEEKLY EVALUATION

What principles has the Lord taught me this week? _____

How can I be more faithful in honoring the Lord next week? _____

What changes am I seeing in my attitude towards:
   Food? _____
   God? _____
   Others? _____

LESSON TWO

The Beginning

Date today _____   Weight today _____
                                              Loss (or gain?) _____

Read 2 Corinthians 5:1-10.

   Vs. 9: "... we have as our ambition, whether at home or absent, to be _____ to him."

What pleases the Lord? (Read 1 Sam. 15:22.) _____
_____

   Vs. 10: "... we must all appear before the judgment seat of Christ, that each one may be _____ for his _____ in the _____, according to what he has done, whether _____ or _____."

The Amplified Bible adds this comment to verse 10:

   "(considering what his purpose and motive have been, and what he has achieved, been busy with and given himself and attention to accomplishing)."

DEFINE: Purpose _____
_____
_____
_____

DEFINE: Motive _____
_____
_____
_____

I have dieted before for the following purposes: _____
_____
_____
_____

Some of my previous motives have been: _____
_____

As born-again Christians, our motives and purposes should be based on God's Word. Read Philippians 3:18-19.

"They are _____ of the cross of _____, whose end is _____, whose god is their _____, and whose _____ is in their _____, who _____ their minds on _____ things."

Is your inward motive to be an enemy of the cross of Christ? _____

Read Philippians 2:1-18. There is much to be learned about motivation in this passage of scripture. We need to take the guidelines mentioned here as our model for our Overeaters Victorious program.

Vss. 1-4: We need to be "of the _____ mind, ... _____ in _____, _____ on one _____."

Paraphrase verse 3: _____

Verse 4 says, "Do not merely look out for _____ _____ personal interests, but also for the interests of _____."

List some ways we can do that at OV: _____

In Philippians 2:5-11 we are given a model for our attitudes:
  Vs. 7: _____
  Vs. 8: _____

On in verses 12-18, we find many more models for purpose and right motivation:
  Vs. 12: "Work out your _____ with fear and trembling."

God works from the inside out.
  Vs. 13: "It is _____ who is at work in you . . . for _____ good pleasure."
  Vs. 14: "Do _____ things without _____ or _____."
  Vs. 16: "Holding fast the _____ of life."

In verses 17 and 18 we are told to _____ with each other.

You can see by comparing Philippians 3:18-19 with 2:1-18 the wide differences between motives and purposes. But how do we get to motives and purposes such as found in Philippians 2 when we are still living much in Philippians 3:18-19? The answer is in Philippians 1:6. Write it out here:

_____
_____
_____

Who is going to make the necessary changes in your eating habits? _____

Who is going to make the changes in your attitudes? _____ Who is going to give you new motives and purposes in losing weight? _____

WE ARE LEARNING TO EAT IN OBEDIENCE TO THE HOLY SPIRIT, NOT LEARNING TO DIET!

Read 1 Corinthians 3:10-17.

In this life we are involved in building a temple of the _____ _____.

Vs. 14: *"If any man's work which he has built upon it remains, he shall receive a _____."*

Vss. 16-17: *"You are a temple of _____, and the _____ of God dwells in _____. If any man destroys the temple of God, God will _____ him."*

Why would God destroy those who would destroy the temple? _____
_____
_____

Read Haggai 1:8.

Who will be pleased and glorified when you rebuild the temple? _____
_____

Read Haggai 2:3-9.

What promises can you accept from this passage for yourself? _____
_____
_____
_____
_____

ASSIGNMENT:
1. Have a daily quiet time using the Basic Journal Sheet for the next lesson. Include new insights you have about yourself and your reasons for eating. Use a Bible-size spiral notebook for additional journal entries.
2. Record everything eaten and the calorie value on a Calorie Account Sheet.
3. Pray that God will reveal a goal weight—calories per day.
4. Read chapter 3 in *Free To Be Thin* by Marie Chapian.

Preparation for Lesson Three

BASIC JOURNAL SHEET

1ST DAY _____ TIME _____ REFERENCE: Prov. 4:23-24

God is impressing on me: | I've shared with the Lord . . .

Thoughts I'm having today: _____

2ND DAY _____ TIME _____ REFERENCE: Prov. 4:25-27

God is impressing on me: | I've shared with the Lord . . .

Thoughts I'm having today: _____

3RD DAY _____ TIME ____ REFERENCE: Ps. 103:14
God is impressing on me: | I've shared with the Lord . . .

Thoughts I'm having today: _____

4TH DAY _____ TIME ____ REFERENCE: 2 Chron. 16:7-9
God is impressing on me: | I've shared with the Lord . . .

Thoughts I'm having today: _____

5TH DAY _____ TIME ____ REFERENCE: Col. 2:16-19
God is impressing on me: | I've shared with the Lord . . .

Thoughts I'm having today: _____

6TH DAY _____ TIME ____ REFERENCE: Col. 2:20-23

| God is impressing on me: | I've shared with the Lord ... |

Thoughts I'm having today: _____

7TH DAY _____ TIME ____ REFERENCE: Col. 3:1-10

| God is impressing on me: | I've shared with the Lord ... |

Thoughts I'm having today: _____

WEEKLY EVALUATION

What principles has the Lord taught me this week? _____

How can I be more faithful in honoring the Lord next week? _____

What changes am I seeing in my attitude towards:
- Food? _____
- God? _____
- Others? _____

LESSON THREE

Our Goal

Date today _____ Weight today _____
Goal weight _____ Calorie limit _____ Loss (or gain?) _____

Part 1: Setting Goals—Read Proverbs 4:23-27.
COMMITMENT AND ATTITUDES:

   "Watch over your _____ with all diligence, for from it flow the springs of _____."

TRUTH:

   "Put away from you a _____ mouth, and put _____ lips far from you."

GOALS:

   "Let your eyes look _____ _____, and let your gaze be _____ _____ _____ of you."

ATTENTIVENESS:

   "Watch the path of your _____, and all your ways will be _____."

OBEDIENCE:

   "Do not turn _____ _____ _____ nor _____ _____ _____; _____ your foot from _____."

Our goal is to eat in obedience to God through the power of the Holy Spirit. But we can't even begin to obey until the sequence of this scripture is in operation in our lives.

Commitment and attitudes were touched on in the last lesson. *Truth* is required of us on the Calorie Account Sheet. We must be truthful and record even our worst days. It is a method useful in documenting both our victories and forgiveness received.

Then we approach *goals.* Our goal weight is set by God himself.

   Psalm 103:14: *"For _____ Himself knows our _____."*

Pray and ask God how much you should weigh.

   _____ Goal weight   _____ Calories per day

You are going to have to give your *attention* to this program and implement it in your daily life. As a homework assignment, you will be asked to inventory your kitchen and be in touch on an objective level with your food. Be aware of (1) calorie content, (2) sugar content and (3) nutritional information of each item.

Obedience—2 Chronicles 16:7-9.

"For the eyes of the _____ move to and fro throughout the earth that ____ may _____ _____ those whose _____ is _____ _____."

PRAISE GOD! He wants to help you in your walk of obedience, but that help comes through being completely His. That means our attitudes have to match His will for us. Our commitment to Him has to be complete: our goals His goals, our attention given completely to obeying Him, our obedience in His power. We cannot fail when we give ourselves completely to Him.

Part 2: Holding to the Head—Read Colossians 2:16-23.

"Let ____ man act as your judge in regard to _____ or _____ or in respect to a festival or a new moon or a Sabbath day . . ."

Does dieting *"in the flesh"* lead to *"delighting in self-abasement"*? _____

Verses 20-22 are clear about fad diets and restrictive programs. Perhaps you have been on some of these diets or programs before. As a way of giving these past activities up to the Lord, list the programs that you have tried on your own without Him.

Lord, I give up these ways I have tried in the past to control my weight:

_____   _____
_____   _____
_____   _____

V. 23: These problems and diets have *"the _____ of wisdom, in _____-_____ religion, and _____-_____ and severe treatment of the _____, but are of _____ _____ against _____ _____."*

If you could conquer *"fleshly indulgence,"* could you lose weight? _____

WE MUST COUNT CALORIES TO CONTROL AND INTELLIGENTLY BE IN TOUCH WITH THE REALITY OF WHAT WE ARE PUTTING IN OUR MOUTHS, BUT WE DO NOT LOOK TO COUNTING CALORIES TO CHECK THE INDULGENCE OF THE FLESH. ONLY JESUS CAN AND HAS, IN FACT, DONE THAT FOR US (Col. 3:1-10). If we do not hold fast to Jesus, the Head (2:19), counting calories will only fan the flames of our unruly appetites.

We can have no part of the "dieting-to-eat-again" philosophy.

Our attitudes toward food must be completely changed.

ASSIGNMENT:
1. Have a daily quiet time using the Basic Journal Sheet in preparation for the next lesson. Make additional entries in your spiral notebook of other meaningful scriptures. Include the insight God reveals to you.
2. Record everything eaten with calorie counts on a Calorie Account Sheet.
3. Inventory the food in your kitchen. Be aware of calorie content, sugar content and nutritional information of each item.
4. Pray that God will help you choose foods before you eat.
5. Read chapters 4-7 in *Free To Be Thin* by Marie Chapian.

NOTE:

Have you ordered the next teaching series? Now would be a good time if you plan to continue. Use the form in the back of the book to receive a current price list.

Preparation for Lesson Four

BASIC JOURNAL SHEET

1ST DAY _____ TIME _____ REFERENCE: Dan. 1:1-5; 1 Pet. 1:1-7

God is impressing on me: | I've shared with the Lord . . .

Thoughts I'm having today: _____

2ND DAY _____ TIME _____ REFERENCE: Dan. 1:8; Rom. 8:5-6

God is impressing on me: | I've shared with the Lord . . .

Thoughts I'm having today: _____

3RD DAY _____ TIME ___ REFERENCE: Dan. 1:9; Phil. 1:6, 2:13
God is impressing on me: | I've shared with the Lord . . .

Thoughts I'm having today: _____

4TH DAY _____ TIME ___ REFERENCE: Dan. 1:17; James 1:5-8
God is impressing on me: | I've shared with the Lord . . .

Thoughts I'm having today: _____

5TH DAY _____ TIME ___ REFERENCE: Dan. 1:20; 2 Cor. 5:14-21
God is impressing on me: | I've shared with the Lord . . .

Thoughts I'm having today: _____

6TH DAY _____ TIME ____ REFERENCE: Ps. 27:4, 37:4
God is impressing on me: | I've shared with the Lord . . .

Thoughts I'm having today: _____

7TH DAY _____ TIME ____ REFERENCE: Isa. 30:1-2, 18-22, 25
God is impressing on me: | I've shared with the Lord . . .

Thoughts I'm having today: _____

WEEKLY EVALUATION

What principles has the Lord taught me this week? _____

How can I be more faithful in honoring the Lord next week? _____

What changes am I seeing in my attitude towards:
    Food? _____
    God? _____
    Others? _____

LESSON FOUR

Deciding to Obey

Date today _____ Weight today _____
Goal weight _____ Calorie limit _____ Loss (or gain?) _____

Part 1: Study Daniel Principles. Read Daniel 1 (Amplified if possible).

1. Chosen for the King's personal service (1 Pet. 1:1-2).
2. I have made up my mind that I will not defile myself with disobedience (Rom. 8:5-6).
3. God grants me favor and compassion (Phil. 1:6, 2:13).
4. God gives me knowledge and intelligence in every branch of literature and wisdom. He will teach me which foods are good and which are bad for me (James 1:5-8).
5. I have entered the King's personal service (2 Cor. 5:14-21).

Part 2: Desires/Actions Worksheet

Psalm 27:4: "One thing _____ _____ _____ from the Lord, that _____ _____ _____."

Are you asking God to take your appetite and then seeking a fat life through your behavior? Our desires and actions need to come into agreement. We can't ask to lose weight and still eat beyond our calorie limit.

Psalm 37:4: "_____ yourself also in the _____; and He will _____ you the _____ of your heart."

DEFINE: "Delight" _____
_____
_____
_____

How do you plan to delight in the Lord in your eating? _____
_____
_____
_____
_____

Let's confirm our *desires* with our *actions*!

Part 3: The Battle—Read Isaiah 30.

1. Forsaking rebellious ways and entering into obedience.
   What is your most difficult problem with rebellion concerning food?
   Vss. 1-2: _____

2. Look what happens when you draw on the graciousness of the Lord. How do you let God fight the battle for you?
   Vs. 15: _____

3. Listening to the voice of the Lord. Can you hear Him?
   Vss. 18-22: _____

4. Victory! Who is sitting on the hill playing the tambourine?
   Vs. 32: _____

ASSIGNMENT:

1. Daily quiet time with scriptures, using Basic Journal Sheet for next lesson.
2. Complete a Calorie Account Sheet. Stay within your limit.
3. Prepare a Desires/Actions Worksheet.
4. Read chapters 8-11 in *Free To Be Thin* by Marie Chapian.

Desires/Actions Worksheet

Psalm 37:4: *"Delight yourself in the Lord, and He will give you the desires of your heart."*

DESIRES	ACTIONS
Ps. 27:4 *"One thing have I desired from the Lord . . .*	*. . . that will I seek after."*
Date	Date

Preparation for Lesson Five

BASIC JOURNAL SHEET

1ST DAY _____ TIME ____ REFERENCE: Ps. 119:1, 92
God is impressing on me: | I've shared with the Lord . . .

Thoughts I'm having today: _____

2ND DAY _____ TIME ____ REFERENCE: Ps. 119:9-16
God is impressing on me: | I've shared with the Lord . . .

Thoughts I'm having today: _____

3RD DAY _____ TIME ____ REFERENCE: Ps. 119:33-35
God is impressing on me: | I've shared with the Lord . . .

Thoughts I'm having today: _____

4TH DAY _____ TIME ____ REFERENCE: Ps. 119:65-72
God is impressing on me: | I've shared with the Lord . . .

Thoughts I'm having today: _____

5TH DAY _____ TIME ____ REFERENCE: Ps. 119:105-112
God is impressing on me: | I've shared with the Lord . . .

Thoughts I'm having today: _____

6TH DAY _____ TIME ____ REFERENCE: Ps. 119:57-59
God is impressing on me: | I've shared with the Lord . . .

Thoughts I'm having today: _____

7TH DAY _____ TIME ____ REFERENCE: Gal. 3:23-25
God is impressing on me: | I've shared with the Lord . . .

Thoughts I'm having today: _____

WEEKLY EVALUATION

What principles has the Lord taught me this week? _____

How can I be more faithful in honoring the Lord next week? _____

What changes am I seeing in my attitude towards:
   Food? _____
   God?_____
   Others? _____

LESSON FIVE

The Benefits of the Law

Date today _____   Weight today _____
Goal weight _____ Calorie limit _____   Loss (or gain?) _____

Part 1: Psalm 119

Law is defined in Psalm 119:1 (Amplified) as:

"*the whole of God's revealed will.*"

Keeping in mind the above definition, what then is the "*law*" for you concerning food and your eating habits?

_____
_____
_____
_____

Vss. 9-16: How can a young man keep his way pure?

_____
_____

List five ways to keep our lives in accordance with the Word:
1. _____
2. _____
3. _____
4. _____
5. _____

Then you will delight in the way God is teaching you to eat. You will be able to remember the Word when you need it most. In times of trouble and temptation, when you need comfort and encouragement, you will be able to draw from the Word that has been rooted and planted in your heart.

Vss. 33-35: "*Teach me (_____), O Lord, the _____ of ____ statutes, and ____ _____ it to the end. Give me _____, that I may observe Thy law, and keep it with all my _____. _____ me walk in the path of _____ _____, for I _____ in it.*"

When we understand what God is trying to do in us, we can more readily accept what He is doing in our lives. Pray for understanding into the ways of God that concern you.

Vss. 65-72: "_____ me good _____ and _____, for I believe in Thy commandments."

Paraphrase verse 67: _____

Paraphrase verse 71: _____

Because I am fat, I come quickly to the teaching concerning overeating and discipline. I arrive at the maturity held out to me from the Lord faster than if I did not gain weight so easily.

Vs. 71: *"It is good for me that I was afflicted* [with fat], *that I may learn Thy statutes."*

Vs. 92: *"If Thy* _____ *had* _____ *been my* _____, *then I would have* _____ *in my affliction."*

Read Vss. 105-112:

Vs. 108: *"freewill offerings of my mouth."*

Can you consider your daily restriction of calories into your mouth as a freewill offering?

We can praise God with obedient hearts and behavior, as well as with words and songs.

Vs. 111: When I have fully learned and understood the ways of God concerning me and my weight, it will be a lasting method of weight control, in the power of the Holy Spirit. This victory in Jesus Christ will be the joy of my heart.

Vs. 112: *"I have inclined my heart to* _____ *Thy statutes* _____, *even to the* _____."

How long will we have to obey God in our eating? _____

Pray: From a change that occurs inside me, I will obey you in what I eat, for I have set my mind on your Spirit. I have allowed all attitudes to be examined and changed to fit into your will for me.

I will accept a change in life-style, as far as eating habits are concerned, forever—even to the end!

Vss. 57-59: Review this passage and write out your own personal commitment to the Lord concerning your eating habits:

_____
_____

Part 2: _Galatians 3:23-24_

"But _____ faith came, we were kept in _____ under the _____."

Define "custody": _____

You can even say our calorie limit and the keeping of the Calorie Account Sheet is _protective_ custody.

"Therefore the _____ has become our _____ to lead us to Christ."

Define "tutor": _____

AS WE ARE LOOKING TO JESUS AND LEARNING BY THE POWER OF THE HOLY SPIRIT HOW TO EAT, WE ARE KEEPING OUR BODIES UNDER THE "TUTOR" OF THE LAW (OUR DIET). THE LAW (OUR TUTOR—OUR DIET) CAN SERVE TO LEAD US INTO A DEEPER RELATIONSHIP WITH CHRIST AS FAR AS WHAT WE WILL EAT AND WHAT WE WON'T EAT. ALL THE WHILE, IT IS LEADING US CLOSER AND CLOSER TO WALKING IN COMPLETE OBEDIENCE CONCERNING THE FOOD WE PUT INTO OUR MOUTHS, EATING COMPLETELY IN THE SPIRIT (vs. 25).

ASSIGNMENT:
1. Daily quiet time with the Lord. Use Basic Journal Sheet for next lesson.
2. Complete a Calorie Account Sheet. Stay within your limit.
3. Use "What I Give Up & What I Receive by Giving Up" worksheet as a tool to help get the battle out of the mind.
4. Do a word study on "long-suffering" and "self-control," using dictionary and concordance.
5. Read chapters 13-14 in _Free To Be Thin_ by Marie Chapian.

Give-Up Sheet

(OR "What I Give Up & What I Receive by Giving Up" Worksheet)

Hebrews 12:1 "... *let us strip off and throw aside every encumbrance.*"

WHAT I GAVE UP	HOW I GAVE IT UP	WHAT I RECEIVED
Date	Date	Date

Preparation for Lesson Six

BASIC JOURNAL SHEET

1ST DAY _____ TIME ____ REFERENCE: Gal. 5:22-23

God is impressing on me: | I've shared with the Lord . . .

Thoughts I'm having today: _____

2ND DAY _____ TIME ____ REFERENCE: 1 Cor. 9:24-26

God is impressing on me: | I've shared with the Lord . . .

Thoughts I'm having today: _____

3RD DAY _____ TIME ____ REFERENCE: 1 Cor. 9:27
God is impressing on me: | I've shared with the Lord . . .

Thoughts I'm having today: _____

4TH DAY _____ TIME ____ REFERENCE: Heb. 6:15
God is impressing on me: | I've shared with the Lord . . .

Thoughts I'm having today: _____

5TH DAY _____ TIME ____ REFERENCE: Col. 1:9
God is impressing on me: | I've shared with the Lord . . .

Thoughts I'm having today: _____

6TH DAY _____ TIME ____ REFERENCE: Col. 1:10
God is impressing on me: | I've shared with the Lord . . .

Thoughts I'm having today: _____

7TH DAY _____ TIME ____ REFERENCE: Col. 1:11
God is impressing on me: | I've shared with the Lord . . .

Thoughts I'm having today: _____

WEEKLY EVALUATION

What principles has the Lord taught me this week? _____

How can I be more faithful in honoring the Lord next week? _____

What changes am I seeing in my attitude towards:
    Food? _____
    God? _____
    Others? _____

LESSON SIX

Walking in His Will

Date today _____ Weight today _____
Goal weight _____ Calorie limit _____ Loss (or gain?) _____

Part 1: Long-suffering and Self-control

Define "self-control": _____
_____
_____
_____
_____
_____

Define "long-suffering": _____
_____
_____
_____
_____

Study 1 Corinthians 9:24-27.

"Everyone who competes in the games exercises _____-_____ in all _____."

"_____ buffet _____ body and make it my slave . . ."

Define "buffet" as it applies to your eating habits: _____
_____
_____

Self-control, while it is a fruit of the Holy Spirit, is something *YOU* exercise, with God's enabling power, for yourself.

Hebrews 6:15: *"And thus, having _____ _____, he _____ the promise."*

WHEN WE HAVE THE FRUITS OF THE HOLY SPIRIT, *SELF-CONTROL* AND *LONG-SUFFERING*, WORKING TOGETHER AT THE SAME TIME IN OUR LIVES, WE HAVE AN UNBEATABLE COMBINATION. TRY TO IDENTIFY THOSE TIMES OF WEAKNESS AND DISCOVER WHICH OF THE TWO YOU ARE NOW DRAWING ON.

Part 2: Colossians 1:1-18.

Verse 9: "... be _____ with the _____ of His _____ in all _____ _____ and _____."

Verse 10 lists three things to do: *"So that you may* _____ _____ _____ _____ _____ _____ _____ _____:

1. *"To* _____ *Him in all respects."*
2. *"*_____ _____ *in every good* _____.*"*
3. *"*_____ *in the* _____ *of God."*

Verse 11 gives reasons why; list two:

1. *"Strengthened with* _____ _____, *according to* _____ *glorious might.*
2. *"Attaining all* _____ *and patience;* _____ *giving* _____ *to the* _____.*"*

"GOD'S WILL FOR ME TODAY" worksheet is a tool for planning your day and setting goals—and for receiving spiritual wisdom and understanding for why God wants you to do His will.

Part 3: **"God's Will for Me Today" Chart** *(sample)*

TODAY (Date)	GOD'S WILL FOR ME (What to do)	SPIRITUAL WISDOM & UNDERSTANDING (Why)
	Stay faithful on my diet. Be responsible in what I eat. Fill in my Calorie Account Sheet daily.	To get back the communication between Him and me that brings us so close together and which overeating seems to cut off.
	Start today to take off that last 20 lbs.	To glorify Him and be a witness of His power in my life.
	To clean up my house.	To remove frustration from me. (I eat in times of severe frustration, and a messy house frustrates me.)
	To sew something to wear.	To give me some fun and relaxation, a degree of busyness and a sense of accomplishment. (I tend to eat when I feel bored or useless.)

ASSIGNMENT:

1. Daily quiet time with the Lord. Use Basic Journal Sheet for the next lesson.
2. Complete a Calorie Account Sheet. Stay within your limit.
3. Do a "God's Will for Me" chart.
4. Read chapter 12 in *Free To Be Thin* by Marie Chapian.

God's Will for Me Today

Colossians 1:9: "... *be filled with the knowledge of His will in all spiritual wisdom and understanding.*"

TODAY: (Date)	GOD'S WILL FOR ME (What to do)	SPIRITUAL WISDOM & UNDERSTANDING (Why)

Preparation for Lesson Seven

BASIC JOURNAL SHEET

1ST DAY _____ TIME ____ REFERENCE: Eph. 1:3-8
God is impressing on me: | I've shared with the Lord . . .

Thoughts I'm having today: _____

2ND DAY _____ TIME ____ REFERENCE: Eph. 1:9-16
God is impressing on me: | I've shared with the Lord . . .

Thoughts I'm having today: _____

3RD DAY _____ TIME ____ REFERENCE: 1 Cor. 1:30
God is impressing on me: | I've shared with the Lord . . .

- -

Thoughts I'm having today: _____
_____
_____

4TH DAY _____ TIME ____ REFERENCE: Rom. 12:1-2
God is impressing on me: | I've shared with the Lord . . .

- -

Thoughts I'm having today: _____
_____
_____

5TH DAY _____ TIME ____ REFERENCE: Gal. 5:16
God is impressing on me: | I've shared with the Lord . . .

- -

Thoughts I'm having today: _____
_____
_____

6TH DAY _____ TIME ____ REFERENCE: Gal. 5:22-25
God is impressing on me: | I've shared with the Lord . . .

Thoughts I'm having today: _____

7TH DAY _____ TIME ____ REFERENCE: John 1:7-10 (9)
God is impressing on me: | I've shared with the Lord . . .

Thoughts I'm having today: _____

WEEKLY EVALUATION

What principles has the Lord taught me this week? _____

How can I be more faithful in honoring the Lord next week? _____

What changes am I seeing in my attitude towards:
    Food? _____
    God? _____
    Others? _____

LESSON SEVEN

Position and Practice

Date today _____ Weight today _____
Goal weight _____ Calorie limit _____ Loss (or gain?) _____

Part 1: Read Ephesians 1:3-16.

In Christ we have—
Vs. 3: _____
Vs. 4: We were _____
Vs. 5: _____
Vs. 6: _____
Vs. 7: _____
Vs. 8: _____
Vs. 9: _____
Vs. 11: _____
Vs. 12: We are _____
Vs. 13: _____
Vs. 14: We are _____

1 Corinthians 1:30. Because we had in ourselves nothing, Jesus became for us:
"_____, _____, _____, _____,
_____."

Part 2: Position and Practice

In the light of scripture, which is reality, we have everything we need for a truly victorious life. We have justification, sanctification, and perfection (1 Cor. 1:30). We have been told in Ephesians 1:3:

> *"Blessed be the God and Father of our Lord Jesus Christ, who has blessed us with every spiritual blessing in the heavenly places in Christ. . . ."*

In Ephesians 2:6 we find a similar statement, that we have been placed in Jesus, seated in the heavenlies with Him. How can it be then that we sometimes don't experience this "heavenly" life moment by moment?

As Christians we are to "grow up" in Christ. We are constantly maturing. We get discouraged when we focus more on the day-to-day progress with its momentary struggles and perhaps even defeats than on our actual position in Christ. If you were to graph your progress, you would see that the lessons learned from each struggle and failure can, if you let it have its full work, bring you ever closer to the fullness of your position in Christ. God has planned a way to bring us out of struggles into victory, ever closer to Jesus and the potential life of overcoming that is promised to all who believe in Him. It is called *repentance*—a simple process of confession of sin and turning away from that sin to go on with Him; a constant yielding and surrendering to God in the power of the Holy Spirit. The Holy Spirit enables us to walk more and more victoriously to the extent we daily yield to Him. Let's look at a diagram.

OUR UNION WITH CHRIST—SEATED IN THE HEAVENLIES (Eph. 1:3; 2:6)

Positional justification, sanctification, perfection (1 Cor. 1:30)

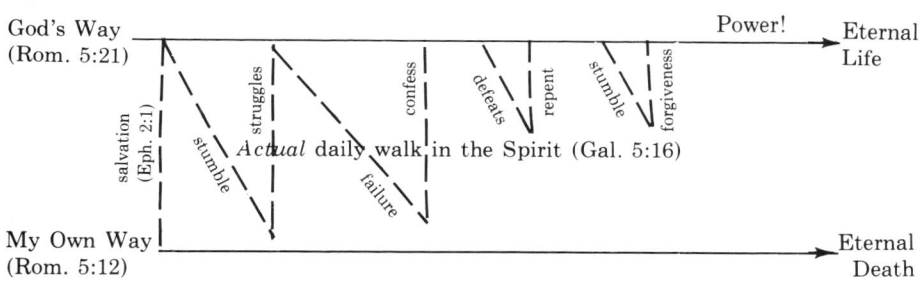

By reckoning ourselves dead to sin and alive to God through the Cross of Christ (Rom. 6:11) and by dying daily (1 Cor. 15:31), the Holy Spirit enables us to have victory over sin and self, over old habits of thinking and doing and reacting.

Keeping in clear focus our POSITION in Christ while living out the day-by-day experiences (the struggles, etc.) helps us to become victorious and helps us to walk in power.

You are secure in Jesus. Your day-by-day struggles do not touch your position in Christ; even though many times it feels like it, your position in Christ remains the same. If you have accepted Him as your Savior, you *are* seated in the heavenly places with Him. Look at the scripture and begin now to focus on your position in Jesus. Then your day-by-day experiences will take on proper perspective and you will experience hope instead of despair and move into victory instead of defeat.

Galatians 5:22-25:

"Those who _____ to _____ _____ have _____ the flesh with its _____ and _____."

1 John 1:7-10:

"... the blood of Jesus His Son _____ _____ us from all sin ... "

1 John 1:9. When does this take place?

"If we _____ our sins, He is faithful and righteous to _____ us our sins and to _____ us from all _____."

Confession! Truth! Keys to Victory!

ASSIGNMENT:
1. Daily quiet time with the Lord. Record special verses in a journal.
2. Complete a Calorie Account Sheet. Stay within your limit.
3. Read chapters 15-16 in *Free To Be Thin* by Marie Chapian.
4. Finish reading *Free To Be Thin*.

CALORIE ACCOUNT SHEET (Sample)

NAME _____ _____ WEEK OF _____ TO _____

Week's Beginning Weight _____ Calorie Limit _____ Starting Weight _____ Goal Weight _____ Week's Ending Weight _____

	1st Day		2nd Day		3rd Day		4th Day		5th Day		6th Day		7th Day	
	Portion	Cal.	Portion	Cal.	Portion	Cal.	Portion	Cal.	Portion	Cal.	Portion	Cal.	Portion	Cal.
MORNING														
total														
MIDDAY														
total														
EVENING														
total														
Daily total														

Books by Neva Coyle:

Free To Be Thin, w/Marie Chapian, a successful weight-loss plan which links learning how to eat with how to live

There's More To Being Thin Than Being Thin, w/Marie Chapian, focusing on the valuable lessons learned on the *journey* to being thin

Living Free, her personal testimony

Daily Thoughts on Living Free, a devotional

Scriptures for Living Free, a counter-top display book of Scriptures to accompany the devotional

Free To Be Thin Cookbook, a collection of tasty, nutritious recipes complete with the calorie content of each

Free To Be Thin Leader's Kit, a step-by-step guide for organizing and leading an Overeaters Victorious group, including five cassete tapes of instruction

Free To Be Thin Daily Planner, a three-month planner for recording daily thoughts, activities and calorie intake

Tape Albums and Study Guides by Neva Coyle:

(The study guides come with the tape albums but may also be ordered separately.)

A Seminar on Living Free (four cassettes) A recording of her seminar in which she shares the principles that have helped her break free from a life of misery and self-satisfaction
Living Free Study Guide, to accompany the tape album

Free To Be Thin (seven cassettes) Victory, Weight-loss, Deliverance
Free To Be Thin Study Guide No. 1, Getting Started, to be used with the book by the same title, and/or the tape album

Discipline (four cassettes) A Program for Spiritual Fitness
Free To Be Thin Study Guide No. 2, Discipline, to be used with the book by the same title, and/or the tape album

Abiding (four cassettes) Honesty in Relationships
Abiding Study Guide

Freedom (four cassettes) Escape from the Ordinary
Freedom Study Guide

Diligence (four cassettes) Overcoming Discouragement
Diligence Study Guide

Obedience (four cassettes) Developing a Listening Heart
Obedience Study Guide

Free To Be Thin Aerobics, available in LP record album with booklet, or cassette tape album with booklet

Detach here

For information regarding OVEREATERS VICTORIOUS and for current price lists on other materials, send a business-size, stamped, self-addressed envelope to Overeaters Victorious, Inc., P.O. Box 179, Redlands, CA 92373.

If you would like to receive special mailings concerning Overeaters Victorious seminars in your area, fill out the form below. (*Allow four weeks.*)

⌐ Name _____

Address _____

└ City/State _____ Zip _____ ⌐ Please print or type.